The Military Diet:
Easy Lessons For Fast And Healthy Weight Loss

Disclamer: All photos used in this book, including the cover photo were made available under a Attribution-NonCommercial-ShareAlike 2.0 Generic and sourced from Flickr

Table of Contents

Introduction: Get Ready for Boot Camp!

The military diet is a strict regimen that has you following rigid meal plans that are designed to help you maximize your weight loss over a short period of time.

Similar to other low calorie diets this regimen calls for participants to consume as little as 1000 calories a day for the first few days. These first few weeks of adjusting to such a low calorie routine is probably the hardest part of the diet and an aspect that I like to call (fittingly enough) "Boot Camp".

But even these low calorie restricted days may not be as bad as you think. Because due to the ingenious design of this program within that finite amount of calorie consumption you will be amazed to find recommendations of hot dogs, tuna, toast and even vanilla ice cream as fat burning food alternative (Yes, I said ice cream).

The toast alone was enough to get me hooked on this diet. Because I'm right there with Oprah when I say I love bread!

And even though so many of those calorie counting diets recommend the complete eradication of bread, the military diet finds a way for you to have all of your aforementioned favorites without a caloric price to pay.

This is all do to the specifically designed "fat burning food combinations" that are given to you to follow, finding ways to use the food you consume to work against fat, and not work against you!

For example, the founders of this diet have discovered that the simple pairing of grapefruit with peanut butter toast can to wonders in helping jumpstart your metabolism and aiding your body to shed calories.

It is through seemingly simple discoveries like this that the Military Diet is able to succeed where so many others fail. And your period of boot camp restriction is only for 3 days, for the other 4 days of the week you can eat more at your normal pace. With such flexibility the boot camp of the military diet should be a breeze!

Chapter 1: Some Military Grade Ingredients

You don't have to be in the armed forces to appreciate some military grade ingredients. In this chapter you will learn exactly what and where to buy the basic necessities you need in order to stay on track for your military diet. You don't have to buy anything fancy for this diet, or anything specialty made, most of what you need can be found at your local grocery store.

Wherever you may go to get your food however, your most important priority is to make sure that your food is fresh. It is a simple rule of thumb, the fresher the ingredients you use the more nutritional value that you will get from the product. If you buy ingredients way ahead of their expiration date, that also means they will last much longer in your home.

So yes, always go for the freshest foods you can find. Along with loading up on fresh food you should also try to get as many common staples as you can such as rice, beans, eggs, milk and butter. Beans in particular are very important parts of any diet and this is especially the case with a military one. Beans are a great natural source of energetic metabolism, and you should stock up on a wide variety such as, pinto, garbanzo, chili, and black beans.

Rice is a great counterbalancing ingredient for any meal and butter is integral for many dishes as well. Make sure you stock up on all of these basic necessities. Next to all of these staples of your diet, you should also work to enhance your supply of dairy products. Number one in your dairy arsenal should be skim milk. Surely you have seen that pint of milk at the grocer with the pink lid? Yes my friends, that; is skim milk.

The taste of skim milk is a little less full than that of its whole milk variety, but the savings in calories will be well worth it. And besides, after using it for a while, many learn to love the taste and even come to prefer it to the whole milk variety. I know this first hand, because after drinking skim milk for many years now, and if someone gave me a glass of whole milk, I wouldn't be able to drink it.

After years of skim it just seems to thick and frothy, so as you can see, skim milk is an acquired taste, but if you are serious about losing weight you will definitely get used to it. With your skim milk supply taken care of, the next dairy product you should load into the fridge is a good batch of yogurt.

This metabolism boosting substance is good for your health and will be a mainstay for menu of the meals you will eat on the Military Diet, so you might as well load up on it now. Cheese shouldn't be neglected either, though we need to make sure that we don't use cheese that is too rich or fattening there are many varieties you can use that will not interfere with your Military Diet.

Along with cheese a good brand of light butter should be included in your Military Diet dairy itinerary as well. Besides dairy also make sure to stockpile eggs.

Most people love the taste of eggs, and despite what some may have said about there cholesterol content through the years, eggs are mainly harmless when eaten in moderation. In fact they can be a great boon to your health, as the special combinations of the Military Diet will demonstrate later in this book; because you need military grade ingredients for a military grade diet.

Chapter 2: Starting Your Meal Plan

The most important part of the military diet is setting up a meal plan. You need to be able to gear up your metabolism to get through the rest of the 3 days of the military diet. So let's break it down day by day and meal by meal.

 For your first day, you should have solid meals consisting of some strong staples to help gird your metabolism and stamina. Here are a few suggestions for the first meal of the day!

Basic Military Breakfast

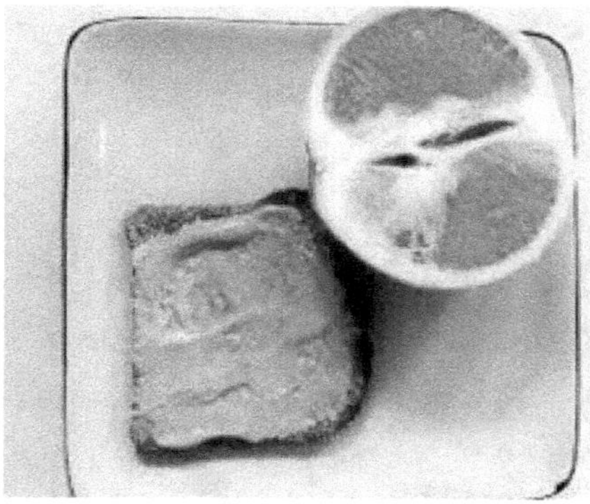

This meal cuts out the trimmings and just gives it to straight. With wholegrain and black coffee you are inaugurating your day with grit and determination!

Here are the exact ingredients:
1/3 slice of Grapefruit

1 Piece of Wholegrain Toast

1 tbsp of Peanut Butter

1 Cup of Green Tea or Black Coffee

This one is a real no brainer. Its basic but good. Just take a Grapefruit and cut off a 1/3 slice and put it on a plate. Now take a plain piece of wholegrain bread and toast it in your toaster.

Add the toast to the plate. Now add your 1 tbsp of peanut butter to the toast, evenly distributing the peanut butter to the bread. You can then make yourself a cup of green tea or black coffee (whichever you prefer) and you have yourself a great way to start your day.

Mushrooms and Scrambled Eggs

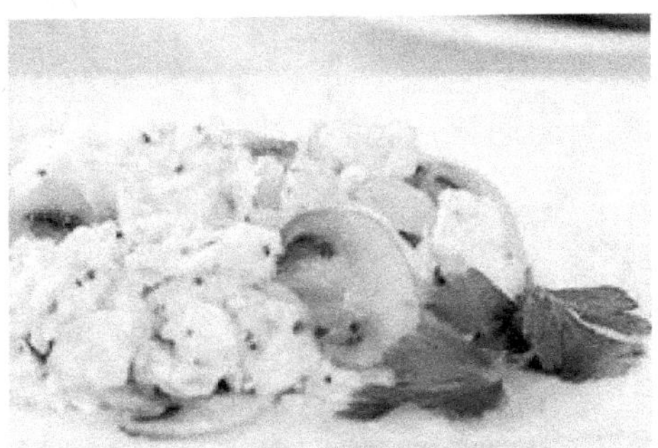

I love scrambled eggs, and I'm sure a lot of you out there do too. Well thanks to the rigid fixings of the military diet you can enjoy this dish without fear. It cuts out the fat and gives you the filling to start your day!

Here are the exact ingredients:

2 eggs

1 tbsp chopped chives

½ tbsp olive oil

½ cup of mushrooms, finely diced

¼ cup of green pepper, finely diced

Layer a frying pan with your half a tablespoon of olive oil and place it over medium heat. Now crack your eggs over your pan being sure to let all of the yolk and egg white fall into place. Take out a wooden spoon and vigorously stir your eggs until the yolk and egg whites are thoroughly mixed together.

With your egg material in place, you can now add your chopped chives, diced mushrooms and diced green pepper. Mix all of your ingredients together for a few more minutes and then turn your burner off. Your mushroom and scrambled egg dish is now ready to eat!

Cheese and Crackers

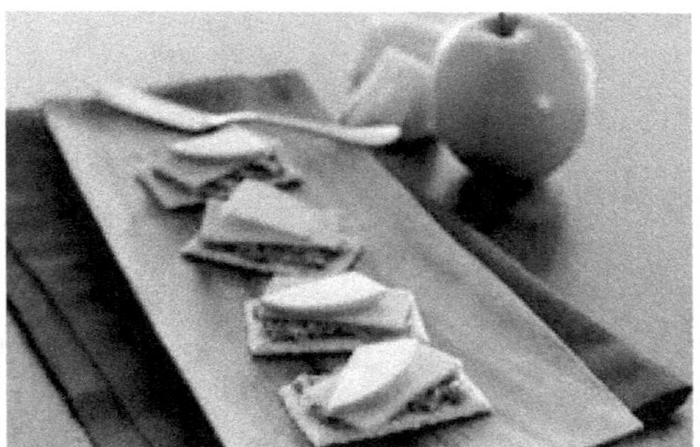

This breakfast is admittedly on the slim side, but with all the calories you save you can eat more later on in the day!

Here are the exact ingredients:
4 regular saltine crackers
1 slice of cheddar cheese
1 small apple

This is a really simple meal, basically just grab yourself 4 crackers and then evenly distribute your slice of cheddar cheese. Then eat your apple and you are ready
to get showered ad ready for your day.

Army Omelets

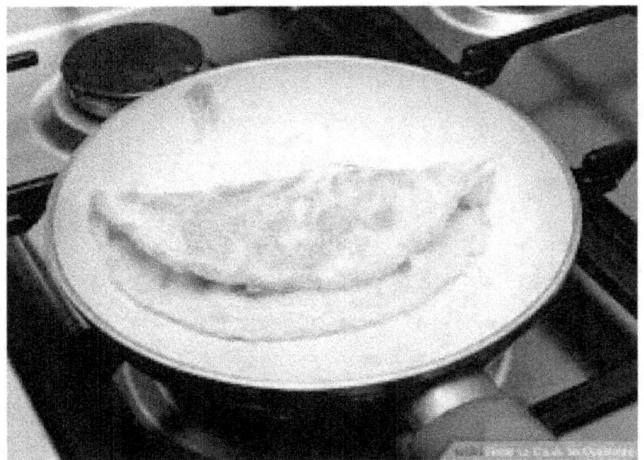

Eggs are great any time of day, but especially in the morning! So its good to know,
with so many egg based recipes, that the military diet is all about the ever incred-
ible egg! Ok then soldier! Just sink your teeth into this Army Omelet!

Here are the exact ingredients:
1 large egg
½ tbsp skim milk
½ tbsp salt

First, crack your egg over a medium skillet, letting the yolk and egg white settled
to the bottom of the pan. Now add your half a tbsp of skim milk and your half a
tbsp of salt and stir these ingredients into your egg. Turn your burner on high and
with a wooden spoon vigorously stir the egg material together for about 5 minutes as it cooks.

Turn the burner off, take the back of your wooden spoon and use it to smooth down the top surface of the omelet. Once the omelet has fully solidified in the pan simply turn the pan upside down over a large plate and let it drop down onto it. This Army Omelet is now ready to be served!

Military Oats

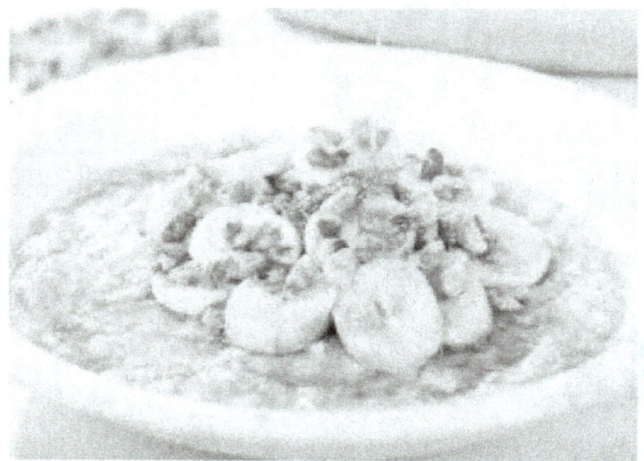

If you're not too big on your eggs and toast; get a load of these Military Oats!

Here are the exact ingredients:

½ an ounce of oats

¼ tbsp of milk

1 tbsp yogurt

½ cup sliced banana

Take out a small mixing bow and dump your ½ ounce of oats inside. Now add your ¼ tbsp of milk and your tbsp of yogurt. Vigorously stir these ingredients together. Now just add your half a cup of banana and you your ready to sow those wild Military Oats!

Chapter 3: Military Mid Day Meals

Once you start getting through your morning you are going to want a light mid day meal to get you through the rest of it. Your mid day lunch break should be something light but filling. Here are a few suggestions for you:

Eggplant Marine Pasta

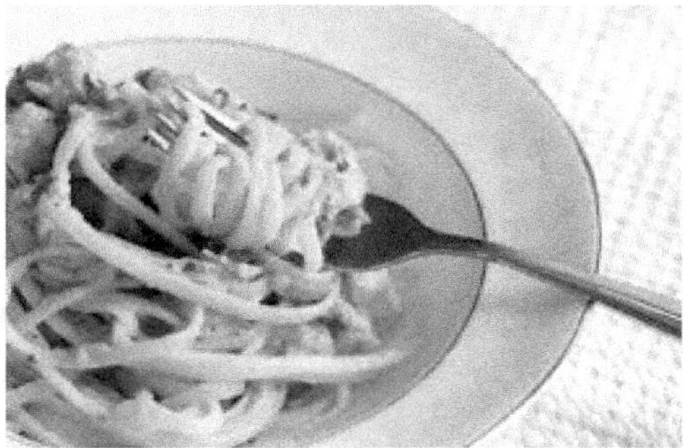

Nothing like some good pasta to perk up your afternoon and with eggplant too boot!

Here are the exact ingredients:

1 tbsp of butter

½ cup of wheat linguini

2 cloves of garlic, chopped

1 eggplant, diced

2 tbsp basil, chopped

½ tbsp olive oil

Take out your eggplant, dice it, and place in medium mixing bowl. Now add your chopped cloves of garlic, chopped basil and your half tablespoon of olive oil. Mix these ingredients together well and set them to the side for a moment. Go to your stove and put a medium sauce pan on high heat.

Add your tablespoon of butter to the pan. Now dump the contents of the mixing bowl into the saucepan and stand and mix the entire contents of the pan while it cooks for 5 minutes on high. Finally add your half cup of wheat linguini, stir for another five minutes, turn your stove off, and serve.

Simple Soldier Soup

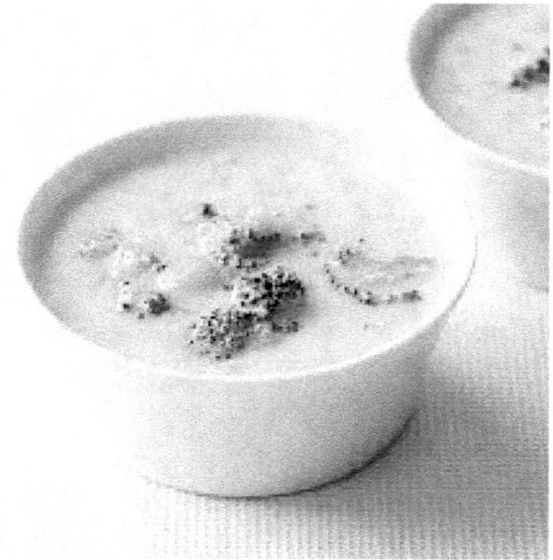

Really there is nothing simple about this soup and it comes loaded for bare, packed with flavor! This soup is a great filler to quench your appetite in the middle of the day. And with ingredients like these it tastes great!

Here are the exact ingredients:

1 chopped onion

1 chopped stick of celery

½ tablespoon of olive oil

2 cups fresh peas

1 cup fresh broccoli

2 tablespoons of soy sauce

½ cup of beef stock

1 cup of water

First put your cup of water and half tablespoon of olive oil to a saucepan and set the burner to medium heat. After this mixture has boiled for a few minutes add your chopped celery, 2 cups of fresh peas, cup of fresh broccoli and half cup of beef stock.

Now mix all of these ingredients together well over the burner for about minutes. Once these are thoroughly mixed just add your 2 tablespoons of soy sauce for extra flair and your Simple Soldier Soup is ready to serve.

Soldier Stir Fir

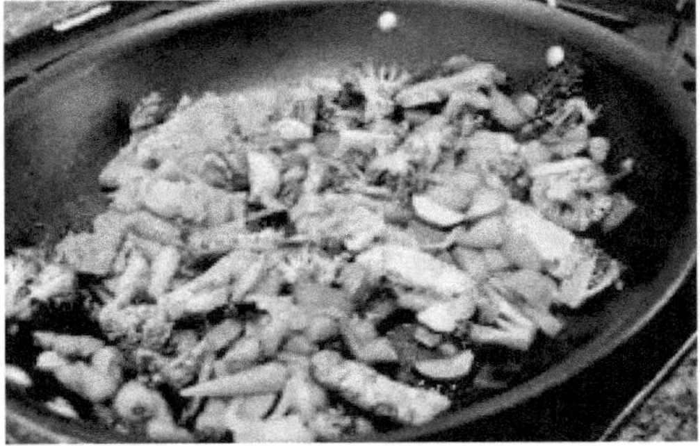

If you love stir fry, you are going to love this addition to the Military Diet.

Here are the exact ingredients:

½ tbsp olive oil

1 green diced green chili

2 garlic chopped garlic cloves

2 cups mixed vegetables

½ cup soy sauce

First coat a medium saucepan with ½ tablespoon of vegetable oil and set your burner to medium heat. Now add your chopped garlic clove, diced green chili, 2 cups of mixed vegetables.

 Let the mixture warm up and then add your ½ cup of soy sauce, vigorously stirring it in as the contents of your pan heats up. Let the whole mixture cook for about five more minutes. And finally, put this majestic stir fry on a plate and eat it!

Uncle Sam's Midday Veggie Roast

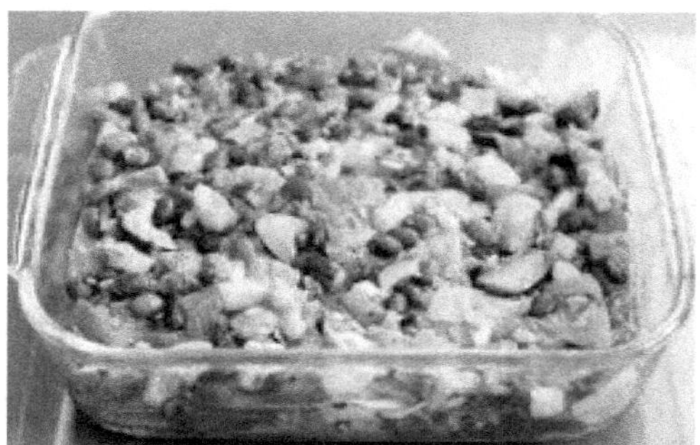

In the middle of the day there is nothing quite like some good roasted veggies! Try this absolutely delicious Midday Veggie Roast!

Here are the exact ingredients:

2 tbsp vegetable oil

3 cups diced zucchini

1 cup diced eggplant

4 cups diced tomatoes

½ cup chopped garlic

¼ cup pepper

¼ cup salt

Set your oven to about 400 degrees and let it preheat for about 10 minutes. Next add your vegetable oil to a baking pan followed by your cups of diced zucchini, egg plant, tomatoes, and your ½ cup of garlic. Mix these around in the pan until they are evenly distributed throughout.

Now place your pan back in the oven and let the entire contents roast for about 30 minutes. After your 30 minutes are up, turn off the oven and place your pan on the stove. Add your salt, pepper and serve up this nicely roasted helping from Uncle Sam!

Chicken Salad

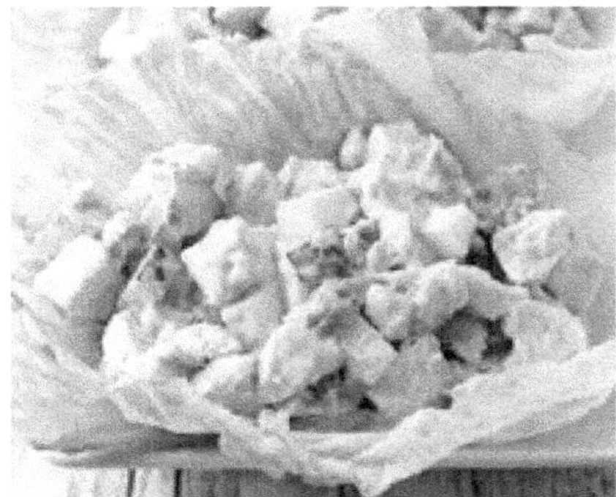

And finally for your midday meal, nothing better than a serving of this tasty Chicken Salad!

Here are the exact ingredients:
5 tbsp vegetable oil
¼ tbsp chopped thyme
1 chicken breast
1 cup of water
1 lemon wedge
1/3 cup of lettuce

To start off, take out a small saucepan, add your cup of water, add your 5 tbsp of vegetable oil and set your burner on high. Let this heat up for about one minute and then toss in your chicken breast. Now let your chicken boil for about 15 minutes.

After this turn your burner off and add your ¼ cup of chopped thyme to the mix. Now set your pan to the side and allow it to cool off. Take out your salad bowl and drop in your 1/3 cup of lettuce. Now add your chicken breast mixture from your plan. Finally put your lemon wedge to the side and your Chicken Salad is ready to go.

Chapter 4: The Soldier Supper

When it comes to supper time, the last meal of the day, you don't want to eat just any slop from the mess hall; you need to have something satisfying and flavorful. In this chapter we will focus on many great dishes that will allow you to do just that.

Fish and Mushroom Platter

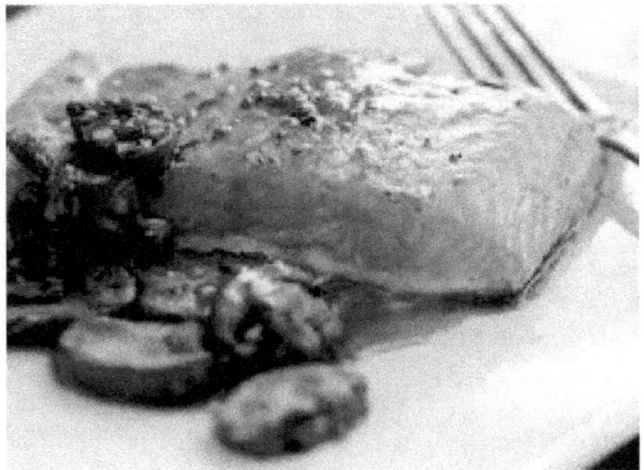

There is nothing quite as refreshing after a long day than a nice platter of fish. Try this recipe and see for yourself!

Here are the exact ingredients:

1 cup of chopped mushrooms

3 salmon steaks

½ cup of vegetable oil

¼ cup thyme leaves

½ cup chopped garlic

2 tbsp butter

1 lemon wedge

This one is good for the grill. So bust out that weekend warrior of yours and set it to medium-high heat. As your grill is heating up, take out your salmon steaks and set them on a clean tray.

Now take a brush and use it to apply your vegetable oil directly to the fish. This is also a good time to sprinkle your ¼ cup of thyme leaves on top of the meat. After doing this place your fish on your grill. With your shrimp (I mean fish) on the barbie take out a medium pan and put it on high heat.

Now add your vegetable oil, chopped garlic, chopped mushrooms and butter to the pan. Stir this mixture while it cooks for about 5 minutes. Turn off the burner, go to your grill, take your fish and transfer them to the pan.

With your fish in the pan take a spoon and scoop up the residual mixture and drizzle it over the fish. Let this marinate for another 5 minutes in your pan. After this, just put your fish and mushrooms on a platter and its ready to eat.

Hungry Hungarian Goulash

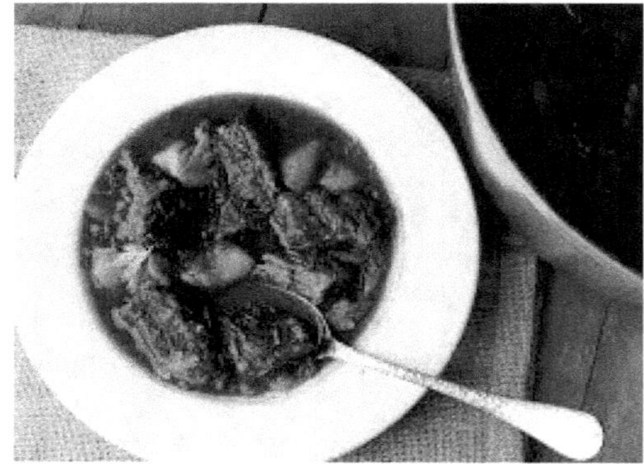

This is a big meal for the end of the day to fill you up right!

Here are the exact ingredients:

1 cup chopped onion

1 cup chopped beef

1 tbsp vegetable oil

2 tbsp paprika

1 cup diced tomato

½ cup water

Start out by frying your beef in a medium saucepan coated with your tablespoon of vegetable oil for about 5 minutes. Once the beef is cooked dump it into a plastic container and put it to the side. Now go back to your saucepan and add your chopped onion and diced tomato, along with your half cup of water.

Begin stirring the ingredients together and let it cook on medium heat for about 5 minutes. Now reintroduce your cooked beef to the pan, add your 2 tbsp of paprika and stir thoroughly for another few minutes. Your Hungry Hungarian Goulash is now ready to go!

Chicken Commando

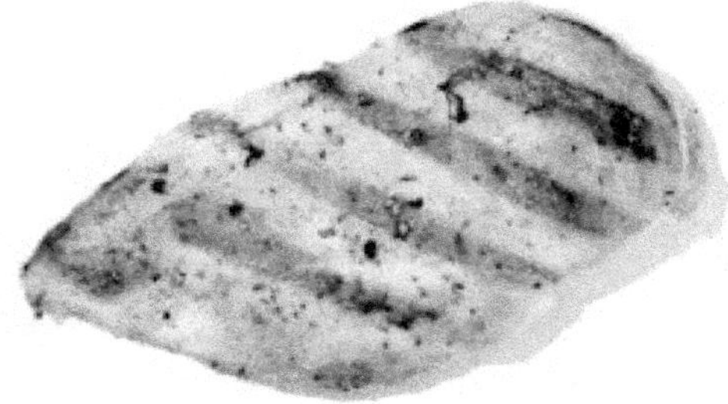

Have you ever felt like going commando? Well what about Chicken Commando? Eat a chicken based dish that has a real command over the appetite!

Here are the exact ingredients:

1 chicken breast, sliced

3 tbsp vegetable oil

3 garlic cloves, chopped

1 tbsp paprika

½ tbsp cumin

½ tbsp oregano

1 tbsp lemon juice

First, put your sliced chicken breast in a small saucepan on high heat for about 15 minutes. While your chicken cooks then mix your 3 tbsp vegetable oil, your chopped garlic, paprika, oregano, and cumin together in a medium sized mixing bowl.

Now add your cooked chicken to the bowl and cover it with either a plastic lid or some kind of wrap. Put this in the refrigerator for about an hour. After your hour is up take out your bowl and sprinkle your tbsp of lemon juice over the ingredients. Your Chicken Commando is now ready for consumption!

Mess Hall Chowder

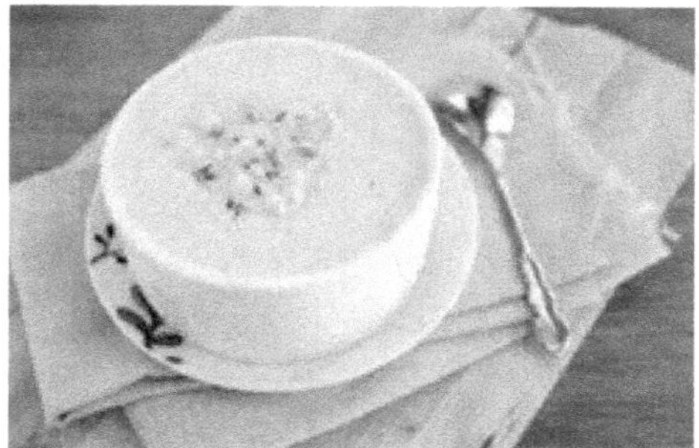

I'm not sure if this dish is like the old mess hall grub or not, but it sure tastes great! I'd wait in line for this one!

Here are the exact ingredients:
1 cup of chicken stock
2 cups of frozen corn
1 cup of chopped onion
½ cup pg skim milk
½ cup of water
¼ of tbsp salt

Put your chopped onion in a saucepan; add your ½ cup of water and put the burner on medium hit. Now add your 2 cups of frozen corn, and your cup of chicken stock.

Let this mixture cook for about ten minutes, stirring frequently. After the ten minutes have passed, turn the burner off and add your ½ tbsp of salt to the mix, sprinkling it on top. This chowder is now ready for the mess hall!

Potato Casserole

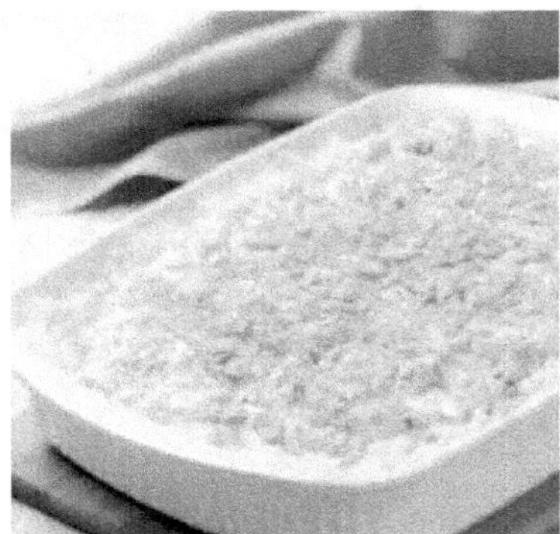

This dish combines two of my favorite dishes for a heart suppertime meal. There are definitely no regrets with the Military Diet when you can eat a dish like this!

Here are the exact ingredients:
2 large tomatoes
3 cups diced potatoes
2 cups chopped onion
1 cup vegetable oil
1 tbsp basil, chopped
3 tbsp parsley, chopped
1 cup water
2 tbsp paprika
1 tbsp pepper
2 cups baked tofu, chopped

Chop and dice all of your tomatoes, potatoes, and onions. Now mix these ingredients together and add them to a pan with 1 cup of vegetable oil. Turn on your burner to medium heat and go ahead and add your cup of water to the pan. Stir the ingredients together and then add your 2 cups of baked tofu. Continue to stir and then sprinkle in your basil and parsley right on top of the mixture.

After this is well blended and cooked together transfer the contents of your pan to a baking sheet in the oven. Make sure that your baking sheet is of oven safe material and prep it for cooking. Now let this cook for 30 minutes on 400 degrees. Take out your pan and sprinkle your paprika, pepper, basil, and parsley on top. This Potato Casserole is now ready for dinner!

Tuna Banana and Vanilla Ice Cream

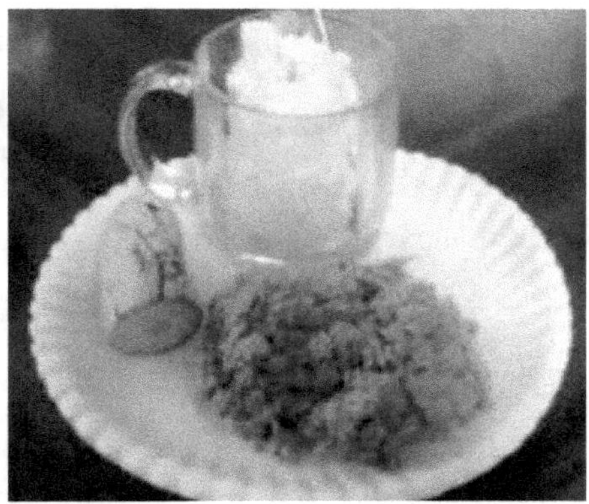

This may sound like an odd combination. But these meal combo does wonders for the metabolism and the waistline!

Here are the exact ingredients:

1 cup tuna

½ banana

1 cup vanilla ice cream

This military meal doubles as a late night snack. Just chop up half a banana and mix it with your cup of vanilla ice cream in a small bowl. Eat this combo along with your cup of tuna. The tuna can be lightly salted and peppered for flavor. Consume this with a large glass of water. This should be your last meal of the day so make it count!

Chapter 5: The Mechanics of the Military Diet

Now that you have seen some of the best recipes of this diet, lets go over just how this diet actually works. The first thing that you need to know—and there is really know surprise behind it—is the fact that the Military Diet is low in calories.

Working on the age old premise that the less calories you consume, the less fat that your body will form. The Military Diet has you maintain a low caloric intake so that you will lose weight.

The other component that the Military diet employs, like many other dieting programs, is that it engages in a form of intermittent fasting. Just like in other diets such as the "5:2" diet the Military Diet works on the concept that while an all out fast of the body, can be bad an intermittent fasting period can be very good.

You see, when people refuse to eat for days on end in a desperate attempt to lose weight in an all out fast, they may lose some pounds but this direct fast will also put their body into a heightened state of alert, causing their metabolism to slow way down.

And like every good dieter knows, a slow metabolism is bad for weight loss! But if you fast or eat very light—as is the case with the Military Diet—for just a few days and then go back to your normal eating routine for the rest of your week, you will be able to lose weight rapidly without slowing your metabolism down.

In fact, everything about this diet is designed to do quite the opposite and speed your metabolism up. With foods that are high in protein, high in calcium, and high in fiber used in consistent patterns that will help raise metabolism as much as possible.

And as mentioned earlier, the diet is actually only three days a week, allowing you to resort back to your old eating habits for the rest of the week, making the commitment to this eating regimen much easier to fulfill.

When I first started the Military Diet it appealed to me right away, because I quickly realized that this was a diet of complete transparency. There was no hidden methodology; it was all right there in my face. I knew what I needed to do, and I had a clear and concise method to do it. Once you know how the basic mechanics of the military diet works, you will want to stick out this weight loss regiment all the way to the end.

Chapter 6: How to Make Sure You Do Your Best

Just following the scheduled meal plans alone is enough for most people to see some real results, but along with following this regimen, there are a few other specific steps you can take in order to proactively ensure your success. First of all you should start every single day with a big glass of water and be sure to drink a nice tall glass of it before each and every meal.

You should also stock up everything you need from the grocery store well in advance so you can avoid engaging in the disastrously damaging "hunger shopping". Now its not quite like the hunger games, but when your stomach is rumbling all the way to aisle 12 it can still be quite a nuisance! You should always wait until your weekly regimen has run its course until you even think about grocery shopping so that you don't lead yourself into any unnecessary temptation at the store.

Another thing you should set in motion early in your day is your daily physical exercise. Although exercise isn't mandatory for the Military Diet to work, it will of course greatly speed the process if you are physically active and the best time to jumpstart your body and metabolism with physical activity is early in the day, shortly after you first wake up.

This workout is also best on an empty stomach, because the emptier your stomach is as you exercise in the morning, the more you will be able to utilize your stored fat as a fuel, and burn it up. In addition to all of these assets to the Military Diet routine, another great boon to your effort in losing weight is to recruit a good friend to share the journey with you.

Having a good companion; whether family, or friend; can prove to be invaluable to keep you on track during this program. I know in from my own personal experience, when me and my wife both tried out this dieting program together we became each others best motivational guide in the process.

 If one of us was about to slip and mess up our diet the other help get things right back on track. Having a good partner with this eating regimen is a great way to make sure you adhere to all of the aspects of the Military Diet.

Taking measurements of your progress is another way to make sure you keep going, because actually seeing the results of your labor has got to be the best motivator there is to any diet! So keep all of this in the forefront the whole time you are sticking to your routine, remind yourself of the inches and pounds you have shed and keep a close eye out as your gain some new room in your old articles of clothing!

Conclusion: In the Army Now!

Just like a crash bourse in the armed services. The Military Diet doesn't mess around with any unnecessary fluff or filler and simply cuts right to the chase. You no doubt picked up this book seeking for just such a diet that would teach you directly what you need to lose weight. Well congratulations my friend, because you did in fact find what you are looking for.

But please let me remind you, this diet will only work if you put in the effort to see it through to the finish line. Like any other diet out there at its core it is ¼ structure and ¾ willpower. Because in the end it is up to you to see it through all the way to the end, so stiffen that upper lip and get down to business soldier, because you are in the army now! I hope this book is helpful in your journey. Thank you for reading!

FREE Bonus Reminder

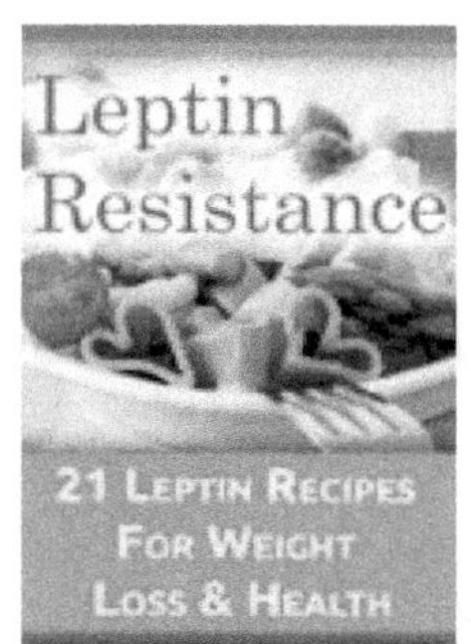

If you have not grabbed it yet, please go ahead and download your special bonus report *"Leptin Resistance. 21 Leptin Recipes For Weight Loss & Healthy Living"*.
Simply Click the Button Below

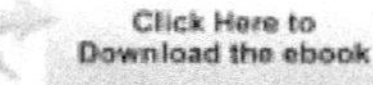

OR **Go to This Page**
http://easyweightlossway.com/free/

BONUS #2: More Free & Discounted Books & Products
Do you want to receive more Free & Discounted Books & Products?
We have a mailing list where we send out our new Books & Products when they go free or with a discount on Amazon. Click on the link below to sign up for Free & Discount Book & Product Promotions.
=> **Sign Up for Free & Discount Book & Product Promotions** <=

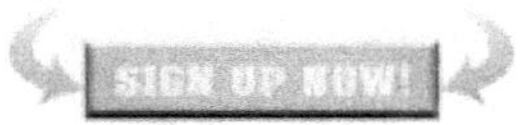

OR Go to this URL
http://zbit.ly/1WBb1Ek

www.ingramcontent.com/pod-product-compliance
Lightning Source LLC
Chambersburg PA
CBHW050711250726
48662CB00002B/959